BASIC FIRST AID HACKS

LAUREEN HOFFMAN

I. Introduction
Chapter 1
Chapter 2
Chapter 3
Chapter 4
Chapter 5
Chapter 6
Chapter 7
Chapter 8
Some first aid measures and hacks that are often overlooked but can be incredibly helpful in various situations.
Chapter 10

I. Introduction

Accidents are inevitable in nature and it is essential that one has the basic ideas to at least help out in cases of emergencies. And that's where I bid you welcome to my book`Basic first aid Hacks": The Ultimate Guide to Basic Life Saving Strategies!

In the course of this book, you will learn, guided and equipped with mind-blowing techniques to respond to emergencies with the use of everyday tools occasionally used items can become of great importance in times of need in cases of Home incidents, Injuries or unexpected crisis

This book unlocks the hidden efficient first aid tips, showing you how to improvise, adapt and react decisively using items that you already have at your fingertips. From turning a scarf into a bandage to using a belt to make a tourniquet, you will learn to harness these basic techniques.

Move with me as you discover how in times of ultimate crisis, Everyday items can come to the rescue.

<h1 style="text-align:center">Chapter 1</h1>

The Power of First Aid Hacks

The principles of first aid are not just based on improvisation; They come with the need for quick thinking, mindset of resourcefulness and the sole belief that one can make a positive impact in the face of danger.

This empowers individuals to become more self-confident when need be. Rather than relying solely on professional responders or well stocked medical kits, you become the first responder. This book teaches you to act swiftly and use what's available to deescalate a situation and potentially save lives in the home scenario.

Its power in problem solving relies on the ability of making use of ordinary items like belts or scarfs as essential tools for survival. It is a knowledge and mindset that turns the simple to extraordinary.

and all in all, gives one confidence when confronted with an emergency. Instead of panicking and being overwhelmed, you will gently assess the situation, identify available resources and apply your newfound knowledge to provide instant help.

This confidence can be a game-changer in high-pressure moments.

The core beauty of First aid hacks is its universal applicability these hacks remains relevant whether at home, work or traveling, they bridge the gap between professional medical care and the critical moments before help arrives

The knowledge gotten from this "Basic first aid Hacks" book is meant to be shared with communities and family to help counter dangerous situations

Instant Injury Evaluation

When I'm faced with an accident, what do I do?How do I react?Who do I contact?How do I help?. These are the questions that everyone should ask themselves as they go about their day to day activities and that's where the knowledge of "Injury Evaluation" comes to light.

"Instant Injury Evaluation" is a critical expertise in medical aid, permitting you to rapidly and precisely assess wounds in crisis circumstances. This comes in very handy when one is a first responder to an accident. The essential steps for performing an immediate injury assessment are carefully explained thus:

Security First: The safety of both you and the injured person should be looked out for firstly. Make sure to properly address any immediate threats or relocate to a safer location. Move away from the scene of the incident if need be.

Really take a look at Responsiveness: Tenderly tap the individual and yell to check assuming they answer. On the off chance that there is no reaction, the individual might be unconscious and not looking so great.

Check Breathing: See, tune in, and feel for indications of relaxing. Place your ear close to their mouth, observe the rise and fall of their chest, and feel for breath on their cheek. On the off chance that the individual isn't breathing or breathing sporadically, check for possible airways blockings before starting CPR assuming you are prepared.

Actually take a look at Heartbeat: Feel for a heartbeat on the individual's neck (side of the neck) or wrist (the part at which most wristwatches are buckled) for at least 10 seconds. Remember to remain very calm while doing so . If trained, begin CPR if there is no pulse.

If excessive bleeding is the case, make use of any clean clothes to apply direct pressure to the injury to control bleeding. Lift the harmed region if conceivable.

Check out the indications of shock, like pallor, fast breathing, or disarray. Keep the individual warm and open to, resting with their legs raised assuming no spinal injury is thought.

Make sure to totally assess the individual from head to toe. Check for blockage of breathing, bleed out regions, swellings, reactions to maybe allergies and try to garner informations about the individual while doing so

Demand Help: Assuming the harmed individual is lethargic or the injury seems serious, call for proficient clinical help (911 or your nearby crisis number) prior to continuing further.

Keep an eye on the individual's condition while trusting that a proficient clinical assistant will show up. When the professionals arrive, make sure to give them every helpful detail and get ready to give extra help depending on the situation.

Having talked about how to react and assess incident situations, we are going to be looking further on how to prevent excessive bleedings and diseases with household items like sugar, honey, duct tape etc

NB: some of these items/procedures may not have conclusive scientific research, but they do come in handy in cases of emergency, so make sure to be wary of that and consult your doctor if needed.

Indeed, even little cuts can bleed a great deal, especially on the off chance that they're in sensitive areas like your mouth or vein region.

With cuts of any size or profundity, the initial step is consistently to apply pressure and raise. From that point forward, there are a few home cures that have been utilized all over the planet to speed blood thickening and prevent the draining from little cuts to major bleeding.

For excessive bleedings , the first step being to apply pressure and elevate the bleeding area above the heart. Apply pressure to the wound for 5 to 10 minutes, then slowly remove hands to see if bleeding has slowed or stopped. If it hasn't, keep applying pressure for five minutes or longer as the case may be. If bleeding still hasn't stopped, call your doctor for advice.

Ice Treatments: For cases where it is an **injury in the mouth, like cut or swelling or even possibly swelling in the face** , applying ice to the affected area might help. It is advisable to apply ice wrapped in a clean thin cloth or gauze.

Sugar or Honey: Sugar and honey draws moisture out of the wound, which can help prevent bacterial growth. They also contain natural antibacterial properties, and they are mostly readily available in our homes. This method can be especially useful for **minor cuts, scrapes, or burns.**

It is important to start by gently cleaning the wound with clean water, cloth and mild soap if available,Pat the area around the wound dry with a clean cloth or sterile gauze.

Then sprinkle a reasonable amount of sugar or honey directly onto the wound. Covering the entire wound surface is important.

Afterwards, you Place a sterile bandage or use a clean cloth over the sugar or honey and secure it in place with tape or a bandage wrap.

These procedures are applicable to burns, scrapes and cuts.

Tea bags: This is mostly used for **stopping Gum** bleedings. If one has just visited a dentist and experiences bleeding from the gums afterwards, adding an unused wet tea bag to the affected area can help stop the bleeding. Brew teabag for some minutes and apply the cool teabag on the affected area. This is possible due to tannin which is contained in tea that aids coagulation. PS: Green teabags are mostly recommended

Salt: applying your wound with some salt might sound like a very painful experience, but it can be quite the opposite. Salt is one of the most important and widely used ingredients. In the case of its importance in first aid, it helps to absorb blood which also helps to dry, close and heal an open wound at a faster rate. This acts as a disinfectant that can even take the toxins out of the infected area to prevent any contamination afterwards.

Petroleum Jelly: In a scenario where it is a **shallow cut,** Petroleum jelly can be used to halt the bleeding. Various cosmetics, like Vaseline products and lip balms, contain petroleum jelly. Petroleum jelly contains a compelling blend of waxes and oils that helps in protecting the skin.

it stops bleeding from small and shallow cuts. Most sports experts in boxing, martial arts, and many fighting sports often use petroleum jelly to treat their wounds. Wipe the skin dry and clean the wound to remove any remaining jelly after the bleeding has stopped.

Bleedings often result from a small cut to a deep, heavily bleeding cut which strikes a serious health risk. Sometimes it may take longer than expected to get medical help. In such situations, to contain the amount of blood loss, you would have to take care of the wound yourself. These tips mentioned above might help you stop bleeding from your wound.

NB: Before you begin to treat an injury, you should identify its severity as best you can. There are some scenarios in which you shouldn't try to deliver any form of first aid at all. If you feel that there's internal bleeding or if there's an embedded object surrounding the location of the injury, immediately call 911 or your local emergency services.

It is equally important to note that

These household remedies are best suited for minor wounds. In cases of severe bleeding or deep wounds, please request professional medical help immediately.

After using these methods, monitor the wound for signs of infection (redness, swelling, increased pain, or pus). consult a healthcare professional at any sign of infection.

Keep in mind that these methods are temporary solutions especially in the case of being a first responder. Professional medical evaluation and treatment are essential for serious injuries or infections.

GOOD HYGIENE MANAGEMENT

It is always important to practice good hygiene especially while dealing with first aid administration. It reduces the risk of contamination of wound and pathogen infestation.

1. Hand Washing:

Wash your hands thoroughly with soap and clean water before touching the injured person or handling first aid supplies. This is the most crucial step in maintaining hygiene.

2. Wear Gloves:

In situations where there is a risk of contact with bodily fluids, consider wearing disposable, non-latex gloves to protect both you and the injured person.

3. Prepare a Clean Work Area:

If possible, create a clean and well-lit workspace to administer first aid. Clear any clutter and ensure the area is free from contaminants.

4. Avoid Cross-Contamination:

Use clean and sterile bandages, gauze, and other supplies.

Avoid touching your face, hair, or other areas that may carry germs.

Do not use your mouth to blow on a wound or an injury. Instead, use a sterile dressing or cloth to provide care.

5. Cover Cuts and Wounds:

If you have any open cuts or wounds on your own hands or arms, make sure they are properly covered with a clean, waterproof bandage or dressing.

6. Maintain Personal Hygiene:

Ensure that your own personal hygiene is at a high standard. Bathe regularly and wear clean clothes.

7. Use Hand Sanitizer:

If soap and water are not available, carry hand sanitizer with at least 60% alcohol content for disinfection in a pinch.

8. Avoid Smoking and Eating:

Do not smoke, eat, or drink while providing first aid. This reduces the risk of contamination.

9. Dispose of Waste Safely:

Properly dispose of used gloves, bandages, and any other waste in a designated medical waste container or trash bag.

10. Keep First Aid Supplies Clean:

Regularly check and clean your first aid kit to ensure that all items are in good condition and free from contamination.

11. Communication:

If possible, communicate with the injured person to understand their medical history, allergies, or any special considerations that might affect the treatment.

Chapter 2

Common household injuries like minor cuts, nose bleeds, head injuries, and their home remedies

Household injuries are inevitable especially when one has a lot of children in the house or in cases of unprotected and sharp tools or areas. It is wise that every individual at least knows how to respond to some cases.

Minor Cuts and Scrapes: The first step to dealing with these types of injuries is to Wash the wound with soap and water to clean it, Followed by the application of an antiseptic solution (hydrogen peroxide or rubbing alcohol) to disinfect it.

Use an adhesive bandage (band-aid) to cover the wound and keep it clean.

NB: make sure to keep children away from all sharp tools like razor or scissors and always monitor them when they make use of one.

Bruises: apply a cold compress (ice wrapped in a cloth) to the bruised area for 15-20 minutes to reduce swelling.

Burns: This is one of the most common types of household injury, especially for those who are mostly in the kitchen. For minor burns (first-degree), cool the affected area under cold running water for at least 10 minutes.

Apply aloe vera gel or vaseline to soothe the skin.

Cover with a non-stick bandage.

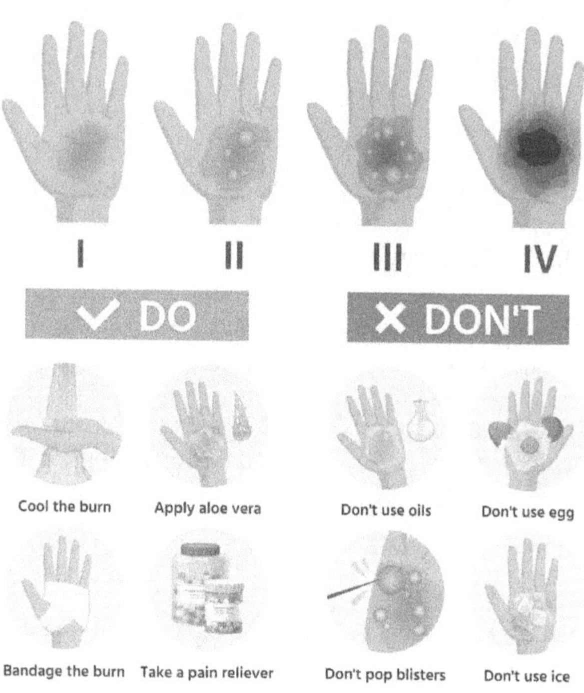

Chapter 3

How to deal with sprains, strains, and fractures with simple techniques, such as RICE (rest, ice, compression, elevation), splinting.

A sprain is basically an injury that affects a ligament, a fibrous tissue connecting bone to bone.

A strain is an injury that affects a muscle or a tendon, which is the tissue that connects muscle to bone.

Sprains and Strains:

It's likely to be a sprain or strain if: you have pain, tenderness or weakness – often around your ankle, foot, wrist, thumb, knee, leg or back. the injured area is swollen or bruised. you cannot put weight on the injury or use it normally.

What to do:

Rest the injured area and avoid putting weight on it.

Apply ice to reduce swelling and pain (20 minutes on, 20 minutes off).

Use a compression bandage to support the injured area.

Elevate the injured limb to reduce swelling.

NB: Over-the-counter NSAIDs (aspirin or ibuprofen) or acetaminophen can reduce pain and inflammation. Talk to your provider before taking over-the-counter (OTC) pain medication for longer than 10 days.

Splinters:

Why is it called a splinter?

Splinter derives from splint, which is a strip or thin piece, a slender piece of wood.

Sterilize tweezers with alcohol and gently remove the splinter.

Clean the area with soap and water, then apply an antiseptic and cover with a bandage.

Nosebleeds:

Pinch the nostrils together and lean forward slightly.

Breathe through the mouth to avoid swallowing blood.

Apply a cold compress to the bridge of the nose.

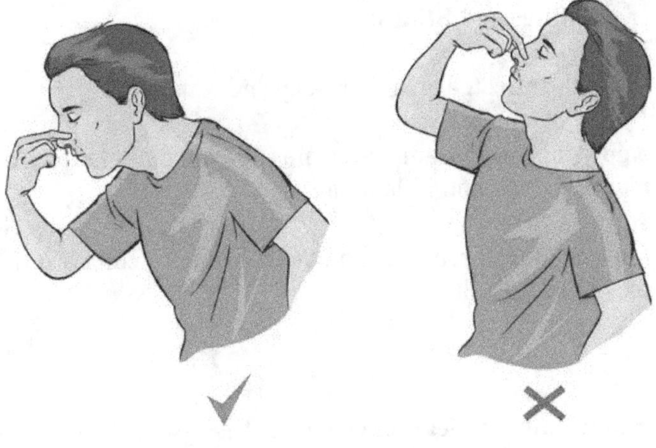

One doesn't need medical help from a medical expert if the bleeding eventually stops, but in cases of severe blood loss, please contact the nearest hospital. Severe cases may include

- the bleeding continues for longer than 20 minutes
- Heavy bleeding and you've lost a lot of blood
- Difficulty in breathing
- you swallow a large amount of blood that makes you vomit

Insect Bites and Stings:

Wash the affected area with soap and water.

Apply an antihistamine cream or calamine lotion to reduce itching and inflammation.

For bee stings, remove the stinger with a credit card or the edge of a knife.

Maintaining a clean environment is essential to avoid insect bites or any bites generally. A clean environment not only helps minimize the presence of pests but also reduces the likelihood of attracting them.

Reducing Breeding Sites, cleaning up crumbs and spilled drinks to avoid attracting them, storing food properly, making frequent use of insecticides, properly cleaning and disposal of waste bins.

An insect bite reduces one to the risk of allergies, malaria, dengue…this is why there is an utmost need for a very clean and tidy environment in order to live a healthy life.

Minor Burns from Hot Liquids:

Cool the affected area with cold water or ice for about 10 minutes.

Apply a burn ointment or aloe vera gel.

Cover with a sterile non-stick bandage.

Minor Eye Irritations:

Rinse the eye gently with lukewarm water for at least 15 minutes.

If a foreign object is in the eye, do not rub it; seek medical attention.

Muscle Cramps:

Stretch and massage gently the affected muscle.

Apply a warm compress to relax the muscle.

Stay hydrated to prevent future cramps.

In addition to these all and staying hydrated, Light exercise, such as riding a stationary bicycle for a few minutes before bedtime, also may help prevent cramps while you sleep.

Choking

Determine if the person is indeed choking. If they can't breathe, speak, or cough, it's a sign of a complete blockage.

Perform the Heimlich Maneuver (Abdominal Thrusts):

Stand behind the choking person and wrap your arms around their waist.

Make a fist with one hand and place the thumb side against the middle of the person's abdomen, just above the navel (belly button) and below the ribcage.

Grasp your fist with your other hand to provide support.

Give quick, upward thrusts into the abdomen, aiming to force the obstruction out of the airway.

Continue these thrusts until the object is expelled or the person becomes unconscious.

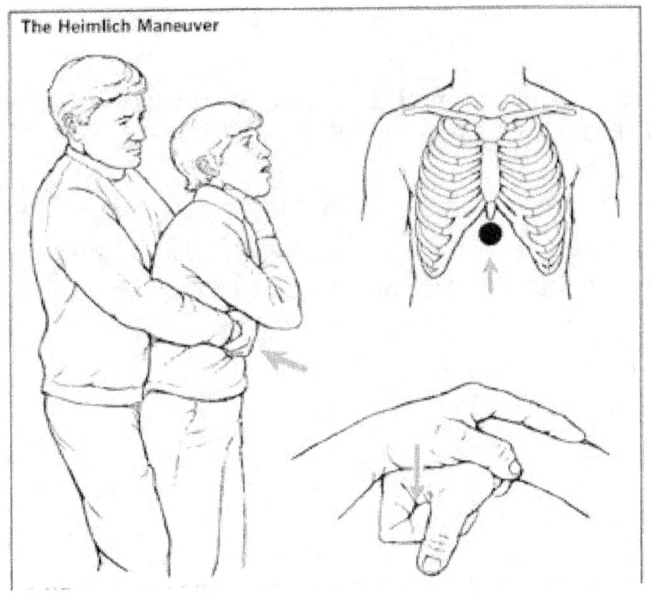

Call for Help: If the person is unable to breathe, speak, or cough, and the obstruction is not dislodged after a few attempts, call 911 (or the emergency number in your country) immediately.

Please note that these remedies are general recommendations and may not be suitable for all situations. If you have any concerns or if the injury is severe, it is always best to consult a healthcare professional.

Chapter 4

How to perform CPR in case of cardiac arrest or drowning.

It is an emergency method used to revive a person whose heart has stopped beating. It can help save a life during a cardiac or breathing emergency.

Situations to Perform CPR:

Unresponsiveness: CPR is required if the person is unresponsive and not breathing normally. Tap the person and shout loudly to check for responsiveness.

Absence of Normal Breathing: If the person is unresponsive, check for normal breathing. If the person is not breathing or only gasping, start CPR.

No Pulse: If there is no pulse, initiate CPR. You can check for a pulse at the carotid artery (side neck) or the radial artery (wrist).

Circumstances Requiring CPR:

Cardiac Arrest: CPR is necessary when someone experiences cardiac arrest. This can result from a heart attack, electric shock, drowning, or other causes. In cardiac arrest, the heart stops pumping blood.

Choking: If a person becomes unresponsive due to choking and cannot breathe, perform CPR after attempting the **Heimlich maneuver.**

Drowning: When someone has been submerged in water and is unresponsive, CPR is required, especially if there's no breathing or pulse.

Severe Allergic Reactions: In cases of severe allergic reactions (anaphylaxis) that lead to unresponsiveness and difficulty breathing, CPR may be necessary.

Drug Overdose: If someone has overdosed on drugs or opioids, leading to unresponsiveness and respiratory distress, CPR might be needed.

Respiratory Arrest: CPR can also be required in cases of respiratory arrest, where a person's breathing has stopped due to reasons other than a cardiac issue.

Things to Avoid During CPR:

Delay: Don't delay starting CPR. The longer you wait, the lower the chances of a successful outcome.

Insufficient Compression Depth:

When performing chest compressions, ensure that you press down at least 2 inches (5 centimeters) for adults and 1.5 inches (4 centimeters) for children. Inadequate compression depth is not effective.

Compressing Too Fast or Slow: Compress at a rate of 100-120 compressions per minute for adults and children. Avoid compressing too fast or too slowly.

Interrupting Compressions:

Minimize interruptions in chest compressions. Stopping for extended periods can reduce the effectiveness of CPR.

Improper Hand Placement: Position your hands correctly for chest compressions, ensuring they are placed in the center of the chest over the lower half of the breastbone.

Over-Ventilation: Don't over-ventilate with rescue breaths. Follow the recommended ratio of 30 chest compressions to 2 rescue breaths for adults.

Hesitating to Use an AED: Automated External Defibrillators (AEDs) are designed to shock the heart back into a normal rhythm during sudden cardiac arrest. If one is available, use it along with CPR as soon as possible.

NB: Endeavor to go for a first aid training or watch some certified First aid videos for better understanding of CPR AND HEIMLICH MANEUVER.

APPLICATION OF CPR:

1. Check the scene for safety, form an initial impression and use personal protective equipment (PPE).

2. Check for breathing, life-threatening bleeding, and other life-threatening conditions if the person doesn't seem to be responding by shouting, tapping, and shouting.

3. If the person does not respond and is not breathing or only gasping, CALL 9-1-1 and get equipment, or tell someone to do so.

4. Place the person on their back on a firm, flat surface

5. Give 30 chest compressions
 --Hand position: Two hands centered on the chest
--Body position: Shoulders directly over hands; elbows locked
– Depth: At least 2 inches

– Rate: 100 to 120 per minute
– Allow chest to return to normal position after each compression

6. Give two Breath
– Open the airway to a past-neutral position using the head-tilt/chin-lift technique
– Ensure each breath lasts about 1 second and makes the chest rise; allow air to exit before giving the next breath
Note: If the 1st breath does not cause the chest to rise, retilt the head and ensure a proper seal before giving the 2nd breath If the 2nd breath does not make the chest rise, an object may be blocking the airway

7. Continue giving sets of 30 chest compressions and 2 breaths. Use an AED as soon as one is available!

Whereas in the case of a child

Look for signs of normal breathing for about 5 seconds. If the child is not breathing or only gasping, initiate CPR.

Place the child on a firm, flat surface.

Kneel beside the child.

Place the heel of one hand on the center of the chest, just below the nipple line.

Place your other hand on top of the first hand.

Keep your elbows straight and use your upper body weight to compress the chest at least 2 inches (5 centimeters) deep.

Perform chest compressions at a rate of 100-120 compressions per minute.

After 30 compressions, give 2 rescue breaths.

Maintain an open airway as described earlier.

Cover the child's mouth and nose with your mouth, ensuring a proper seal.

Give a breath that makes the chest rise visibly.

Repeat these 30 compressions and 2 breaths in a cycle.

Continue performing cycles of 30 chest compressions followed by 2 rescue breaths.

Continue until the child starts breathing, shows signs of life, or professional medical help arrives and takes over.

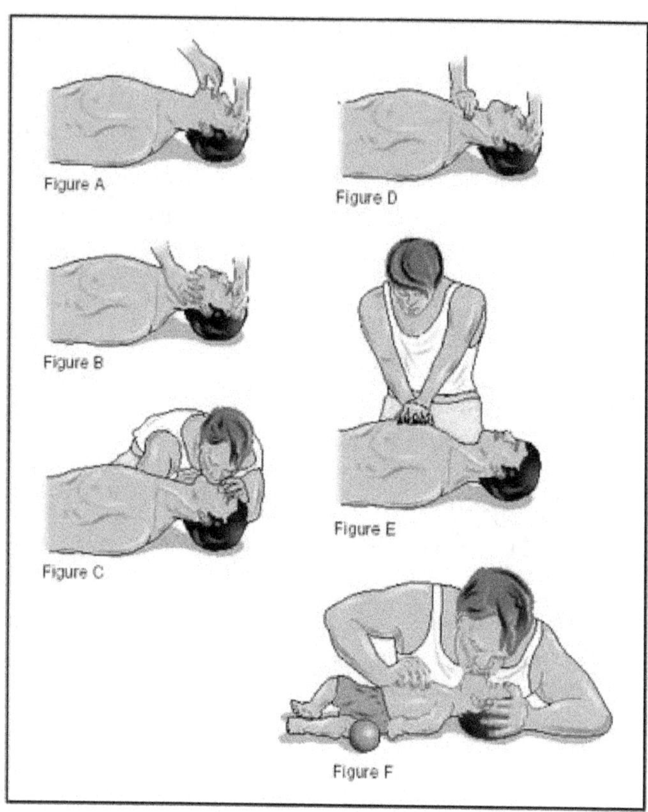

Figure A

Figure D

Figure B

Figure C

Figure E

Figure F

Chapter 5

How to recognize and treat common poisoning cases, such as alcohol, drugs, food, plants, and more.

1. Alcohol Poisoning:

People who get alcohol poisoning may show Signs of confusion, vomiting, slow or irregular breathing, and unconsciousness, an odor of alcohol on the breath, slurred speech and unsteady gait.

Treatment:

Ensure the person is breathing.

Keep them awake and sitting up if conscious.

Do not leave them alone.

Do not try to "sober them up" with cold showers or hot drinks.

If the person becomes unresponsive, call 911.

Home Remedy: Ensure the person drinks water to stay hydrated.

2. Drug Poisoning:

Symptoms vary widely depending on the drug.

Signs may include confusion, hallucinations, seizures, unconsciousness, or difficulty breathing.

Treatment:

Call 911 immediately.

Do not induce vomiting unless advised by a medical professional.

Keep the person calm and monitor their vital signs.

Share information about the substance ingested with emergency responders.

Home Remedy: There is no home remedy for drug poisoning; professional medical help is essential. But it is essential to always crosscheck the currency of drugs before purchase.

It is advised to always stick to a doctors prescription…no more, no less

3. Food Poisoning:

Symptoms may include nausea, vomiting, diarrhea, abdominal pain, fever, and muscle aches.

Onset usually occurs within hours or days after consuming contaminated food.

Treatment:

Stay hydrated by drinking clear fluids (water, oral rehydration solutions).

Avoid solid foods until vomiting and diarrhea subside.

Rest and let your body recover.

If symptoms are severe or prolonged, seek medical attention.

Home Remedy: Consume ginger tea or activated charcoal, but consult a healthcare provider first.

It is advised to make sure of the currency of food when buying canned food and also watch out for any allergies before buying food.

Always cover home cooked meals to prevent external disease infestations

4. Plant Poisoning:

Symptoms vary depending on the plant.

Signs may include nausea, vomiting, diarrhea, abdominal pain, and sometimes more severe symptoms.

Treatment:

Identify the plant and its potential toxicity. Call a poison control center for guidance.

It's very important not to induce vomiting unless advised by a medical professional.

Rinse the mouth with water to remove plant residue.

Home Remedy: In some cases, activated charcoal can help reduce absorption. Consult a healthcare provider for better instructions.

5. Household Chemical Poisoning:

Symptoms vary depending on the chemical.

Signs may include irritation, burns, breathing difficulties, and even unconsciousness.

Treatment:

Call 911 or your local emergency number.

Follow instructions on the chemical's label if available.

If inhaled fumes, move to fresh air.

If skin contact, rinse with plenty of water.

Home Remedy: There is no home remedy for chemical poisoning; professional medical help is crucial.

Avoid applying chemicals like insecticides or repellants in a room or house where people are inside, always make sure no one is in the house during application and give some hours before entering back to the room. During application, make sure to wear a nose mask to avoid inhaling toxic chemicals.

On entering, ensure proper ventilation..

6. Snakebite:

Swelling and puncture marks at the bite site.

Severe pain, redness, and swelling.

Nausea, vomiting, and difficulty breathing.

Treatment:

Keep the affected limb immobilized and at or slightly below heart level.

Remove tight clothing or jewelry near the bite site.

Do not cut the wound or attempt to suck out the venom.

Seek immediate medical attention.

Home Remedy: Applying a cold compress may help reduce pain and swelling.

Leave the snake bite area

Do not attempt to kill the snake to avoid further bites….if you must, move with extreme caution and cover yourself completely.

NB: some snakes are venomous while some aren't, but in order to avoid sad stories, immediately contact emergency care whenever one is bitten by a snake.

It is very essential to keep a very tidy environments that are uninhabitable to snakes

Remember: In poisoning cases, quick action is essential. Call 911 or your local emergency number for professional medical help.

Do not use home remedies as a substitute for professional medical care. Home remedies should complement, not replace, medical attention.

Poison control centers can provide guidance on poison exposure; their number is typically available online and in phone directories.

Always read labels and follow safety guidelines when using household chemicals and avoid exposure to potentially harmful substances.

Important notes:

Activated Charcoal: Activated charcoal can help absorb toxins in the stomach and intestines. It is available in capsule form at most health food stores.

Ginger: Ginger has anti-inflammatory properties that can help soothe an upset stomach. You can drink ginger tea or chew on a piece of fresh ginger.

Cumin: Cumin seeds can help improve digestion and reduce nausea. Boil cumin seeds in water and add freshly extracted coriander juice for best results.

Chapter 6

Heart Attack & Stroke Hints, Allergy & Seizure Swindles, Managing Diabetes Crises, Anaphylaxis Action Plan

Heart Attack & Stroke Hints:

Recognition - Heart Attack:

Chest pain or discomfort, which may radiate to the arm, neck, or jaw, Shortness of breath, Nausea or lightheadedness, Cold sweats, Weakness.

Recognition - Stroke:

Sudden numbness or weakness, especially on one side of the body, Confusion, trouble speaking, or difficulty understanding speech, Severe headache, Trouble walking, loss of balance, or coordination.

Action:

For a heart attack, call 911 immediately.

If the person is conscious and choking, they can chew an aspirin (if not allergic).

For a stroke, also call 911 immediately. Note the time of symptom onset.

2. Allergy & Seizure Swindles:

Allergic Reaction:

Recognize signs like hives, swelling, difficulty breathing, or a severe drop in blood pressure. Administer epinephrine if available, as prescribed, Seek immediate medical attention.

Seizure:

Keep the person safe from injury, placing them on the ground if necessary, Do not restrain or put anything in their mouth, After the seizure, turn them onto their side to maintain an open airway.

3. Managing Diabetes Crises:

Hypoglycemia (Low Blood Sugar):

Recognize signs like confusion, shakiness, sweating, and irritability.

Give the person a fast-acting source of glucose, such as glucose gel, candy, or fruit juice.

Wait for symptoms to improve, and follow up with a snack or meal.

Hyperglycemia (High Blood Sugar):

Recognize signs like excessive thirst, frequent urination, and confusion.

Administer insulin if prescribed or encourage the person to take it.

Ensure they stay hydrated and seek medical help if needed.

4. Anaphylaxis Action Plan:

Signs may include hives, swelling, difficulty breathing, nausea, or a drop in blood pressure.

The person may carry an epinephrine auto-injector (EpiPen).

Action:

If the person is experiencing anaphylaxis, use the EpiPen as prescribed, Call emergency immediately or move to hospital.

Help the person lie down with their legs elevated if they feel lightheaded.

General Emergency Guidelines:

Stay calm and keep the person as comfortable as possible.

Do not give them anything to eat or drink if they are having difficulty swallowing or are unconscious.

Always call for professional medical help in emergencies.

These guidelines shouldn't be used in place of expert medical care; rather, they should be used as first responses measures. In each of these situations, prompt medical intervention is crucial. To be more equipped for every eventuality, familiarize yourself with appropriate emergency response and first aid training as well.

Chapter 7

How to cope with bites and stings from insects, animals, and plants, such as vinegar, baking soda, onion, and more.

1. Insect Bites (Mosquitoes, Bees, Wasps, etc.):

First Aid:

Wash the affected area with mild soap and water, Apply a cold compress to reduce pain and swelling, Elevate the area if possible, Over-the-counter antihistamine creams or oral antihistamines can help with itching.

Home Remedies:

Apply a paste of baking soda and water or a mixture of water and vinegar to the bite to relieve itching.

Rub a slice of onion on the bite to reduce swelling and itching.

2. Tick Bites:

First Aid:

Using fine-tipped tweezers, grasp the tick as close to the skin's surface as possible, Gently pull upward with steady, even pressure, Clean the area with soap and water, Dispose of the tick by submerging it in alcohol, placing it in a sealed bag, or flushing it down the toilet.

3. Spider Bites (Non-Venomous):

First Aid:

Wash the area with mild soap and water.

Apply a cold compress to reduce pain and swelling.

Over-the-counter pain relievers and antihistamines can help with discomfort and itching.

4. Plant Stings (Poison Ivy, Poison Oak, Nettle):

First Aid:

Wash the affected area with soap and cold water as soon as possible.

Apply an over-the-counter hydrocortisone cream to reduce itching.

Take an antihistamine to help with itching and discomfort.

Home Remedies for Plant Stings:

Apply a paste of baking soda and water to reduce itching.

Rub the affected area with a sliced onion or aloe vera to soothe the skin.

6. Jellyfish Stings:

First Aid:

Rinse the affected area with vinegar to help neutralize the toxins.

Soak the area in hot water (104-113°F or 40-45°C) for 20-45 minutes. If hot water is not available, use a hot compress.

Use a credit card or the edge of a towel to remove tentacle fragments.

Seek medical attention if symptoms are severe.

Important Notes:

Avoid scratching or rubbing the affected area, as it can worsen symptoms and lead to infection.

Monitor for signs of an allergic reaction or infection, such as increasing redness, swelling, or discharge.

If you suspect a venomous snake or spider bite, seek immediate medical attention rather than relying on home remedies.

While these home remedies can provide relief for minor bites and stings, they should not replace professional medical care, especially for severe cases or suspected allergic reactions. If in doubt, or if symptoms worsen or persist, consult a healthcare provider or seek emergency medical help promptly.

Chapter 8

How to deal with wounds and infections with natural antibiotics, such as garlic, turmeric, ginger, and more.

Wounds and infections can be treated with natural antibiotics, such as garlic, turmeric, ginger, and more.

Here are some home remedies that may help alleviate symptoms of wounds and infections:

Garlic: Garlic has antimicrobial and antibiotic properties that can help fight off infections. You can apply crushed garlic directly to the wound or mix it with honey to make a paste.

Turmeric: Turmeric has anti-inflammatory and antimicrobial properties that can help reduce inflammation and fight off infections. You can mix turmeric powder with honey to make a paste and apply it to the wound.

Ginger: Ginger has anti-inflammatory properties that can help soothe an upset stomach. You can drink ginger tea or chew on a piece of fresh ginger.

Honey: Honey is one of the most widely studied natural remedies by clinical researchers. It may help heal minor wounds to prevent infections, and is sometimes applied as an alternative to bandages and other skin dressings. Some traditional dressings may also be infused with honey.

Thyme: Thyme has antimicrobial properties that can help fight off infections. You can make thyme tea by steeping fresh thyme leaves in hot water for 10 minutes.

Oregano: Oregano has antibacterial and antifungal properties that can help fight off infections. You can make oregano tea by steeping fresh oregano leaves in hot water for 10 minutes.

Cinnamon: Cinnamon has antimicrobial properties that can help fight off infections. You can add cinnamon powder to your food or drink cinnamon tea.

Echinacea: Echinacea is a herb that has been used for centuries to treat infections. It has antiviral and antibacterial properties that can help boost the immune system. You can take echinacea supplements or drink echinacea tea.

There are some first aid measures and hacks that are often overlooked but can be incredibly helpful in various situations.

1.   The recovery position:

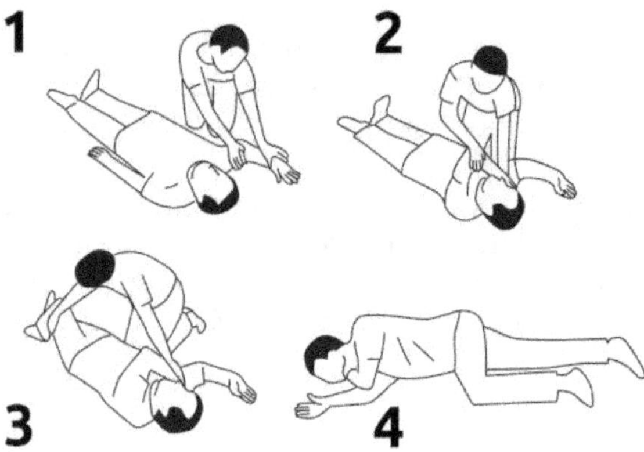

If a person is unconscious but is breathing and has no other life-threatening conditions, they should be placed in the recovery position.

Putting someone in the recovery position will keep their airway clear and open. It also ensures that any vomit or fluid won't cause them to choke.
Even though it's taught a lot, the recovery position is typically undervalued.

It's an essential method for maintaining an unconscious person's airway, particularly if vomiting seems likely. To stabilize the individual, place them on their side with their upper leg bent at a straight angle.

2. Splinter Removal:

It's essential to remove splinters correctly to avoid infection. After sanitizing tweezers and cleaning the surrounding region with soap and water, carefully remove the splinter in the same direction that it entered. After cleaning the wound, use an antiseptic.

3. Sock Trick for Hypothermia:

When a patient has freezing temperatures, cover their carotid arteries with a dry, warm sock. This is a useful first aid tip in cold weather because it promotes the flow of warm blood to the brain more efficiently.

4.Honey for Wound Healing:

Honey has natural antibacterial properties and can be used as a wound dressing for minor cuts and burns. Apply a thin layer of honey to the wound and cover it with a sterile bandage.

5. Tampon for Nosebleeds:

By gently pressing the tampon into the nostril, one can use tampons to control nosebleeds. However if every other approach fails, they ought to be the last option.

6. Ziplock Bag Ice Pack:

For injuries including sprains, strains, and inflammation, make an improvised ice pack by packing a Ziplock bag with ice and wrapping it in a cloth or towel. apply on injury

7. Soap for Insect Stings:

Applying a damp bar of soap directly to an insect sting can help alleviate itching and discomfort. Rinse it off after a few minutes.

8. Onion for Bee Stings:

Rubbing a sliced onion on a bee or wasp sting can help reduce pain and swelling. The enzymes in onions may assist in neutralizing the venom.

9. Tea Bags for Cold Sores:

Because black tea contains tannic acid, using a used, cooled tea bag to a cold sore might hasten the healing process.

It is very essential to note that although these first aid tips and tricks can come in useful in some circumstances, they shouldn't be used in place of qualified medical attention when necessary.

To be adequately prepared for a range of circumstances, it is essential to have a well filled first aid bag, know when to seek medical treatment, and have received sufficient first aid training.

Chapter 10

How to make your own first aid kit with essential items

Container:

Choose a sturdy, water-resistant container to keep your first aid supplies organized and protected. A clear plastic container or a small, portable first aid bag works well.

Essential Items for Your First Aid Kit:

1. Adhesive Bandages:

Various sizes, including small, medium, and large.

Fabric or plastic types.

2. Sterile Gauze Pads:

Sterile dressings of different sizes (e.g., 2x2 inches, 4x4 inches).

Rolled gauze for larger wounds or wrapping injuries.

3. Adhesive Tape:

Medical tape for securing dressings and bandages.

4. Scissors:

Small, sharp scissors for cutting tape, gauze, and clothing.

5. Tweezers:

Fine-pointed tweezers for removing splinters, ticks, or debris.

6. Gloves:

Disposable, non-latex gloves for infection control.

7. Antiseptic Wipes:

Alcohol pads or antiseptic wipes for cleaning wounds.

8. Pain Relievers:

Over-the-counter pain relievers like ibuprofen or acetaminophen.

9. Thermometer:

Digital thermometer to check for fever.

10. First Aid Manual:

- A basic first aid manual with instructions on how to treat common injuries.

11. CPR Face Shield or Pocket Mask:

- For performing CPR while protecting yourself from contact with bodily fluids.

12. Emergency Blanket:

- A compact Mylar emergency blanket for warmth.

13. Elastic Bandage (Ace Bandage):

- For wrapping and supporting injured joints or soft tissues.

14. Safety Pins:

- Useful for securing bandages and slings.

15. Instant Cold Packs:

- To reduce swelling and pain in case of injuries or burns.

16. Sterile Eyewash or Saline Solution:

- For flushing foreign particles from the eyes.

17. EpiPen (if needed):

- For individuals with severe allergies, carry their prescribed epinephrine auto-injector.

18. Any Personal Medications:

- If someone in your household requires regular medications, keep a small supply in the kit.

Additional Items (Optional):

A small flashlight and extra batteries.

Medical adhesive tape or duct tape.

Cotton balls and swabs.

Oral rehydration solution packets.

Pain relief cream or gel.

Resealable plastic bags for disposing of used supplies.

Emergency contact information and a list of any allergies.

Maintenance:

Periodically check the contents of your first aid kit and replace any expired items. Ensure that everything is in good condition and readily accessible.

Personalize your first aid kit based on your family's specific needs and any specific medical conditions or allergies.

Remember, while a first aid kit can be invaluable for addressing minor injuries and emergencies, it is not a substitute for professional medical care in the case of severe injuries or illnesses. Always seek medical attention when needed.

There are several first aid treatments and essentials that are sometimes neglected or overlooked, but they are important for providing comprehensive care in various situations. They include but not limited to:

Eye Irrigation

Neglecting to flush the eye immediately and thoroughly after a chemical or foreign object exposure can lead to serious eye injuries. Eye irrigation is crucial in such cases. A sterile saline solution or clean water can be used for this purpose.

Burn Care:

Properly caring for burns, particularly for more severe burns, is often overlooked. Neglecting burns can lead to complications. First-degree burns (superficial) can be managed with cool, running water, while second and third-degree burns may require medical attention.

Heat Exhaustion and Heat Stroke:

People sometimes underestimate the seriousness of heat-related illnesses. Recognizing the symptoms of heat exhaustion and heat stroke and providing prompt cooling measures are essential.

Fracture Stabilization:

In cases of suspected fractures, ensuring that the injured limb is immobilized and stabilized is crucial. Neglecting to do this can cause further damage and unnecessary pain.

Foreign Object Removal:

When an object is embedded in the skin, it should be removed carefully to avoid infection and complications. Neglecting proper removal can lead to infections.

Anaphylaxis Preparedness:

Having an epinephrine auto-injector (EpiPen) and knowing how to use it is essential for individuals with severe allergies. Neglecting to carry or use it can result in severe allergic reactions.

Stroke Recognition:

Recognizing the signs of a stroke and acting promptly to seek medical help is crucial. Delaying or neglecting to do so can lead to permanent damage.

Applying CPR:

CPR should be administered promptly to individuals in cardiac arrest or those not breathing. Neglecting CPR in such situations can significantly reduce the chances of survival.

Snakebite Management:

When someone is bitten by a snake, proper first aid measures should be taken to slow the spread of venom. Neglecting to immobilize the affected limb and keeping it at or slightly below heart level can worsen the situation.

Preventing Secondary Injuries:

Neglecting to protect an injured person from further harm or injury is a common oversight. Safeguarding against traffic, fires, or falling objects is essential after an accident.

Concussion Awareness:

Recognizing the signs of a concussion, even in minor head injuries, is important. Neglecting to seek medical attention for a potential concussion can lead to long-term problems.

Maintaining First Aid Supplies:

Ensuring that your first aid kit is well-stocked, up-to-date, and easily accessible is often overlooked. Neglecting to do so can leave you ill-prepared in an emergency.

Make a first-rate
FIRST-AID KIT

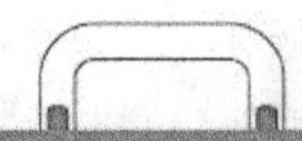

BANDAGES

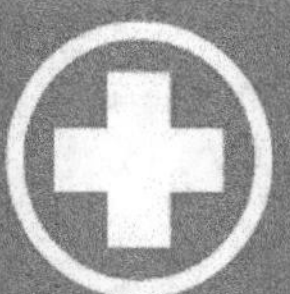

at least 25 bandages in various sizes

Gauze or elastic roll bandage for wounds or injuries that require some compression

MEDICINES/OINTMENTS

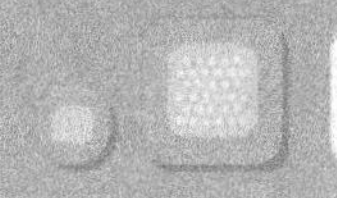

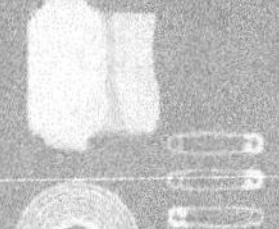

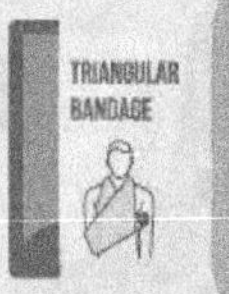

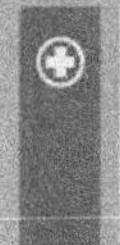
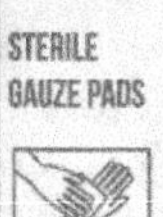

Ointment for itches, rashes and other skin problems

or any other pain reliever

any prescription meds

EQUIPMENT

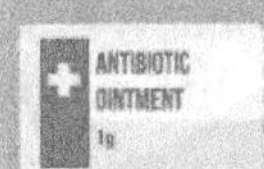

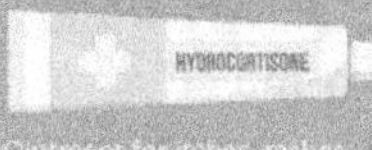

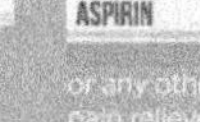

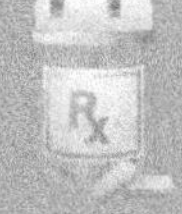

cotton balls or swabs

non-latex gloves

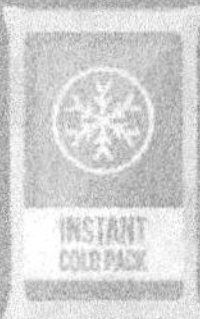
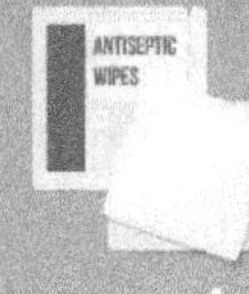
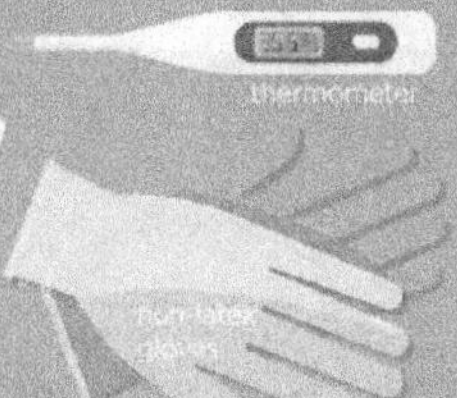
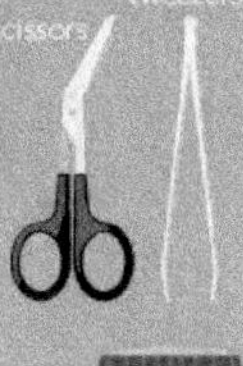

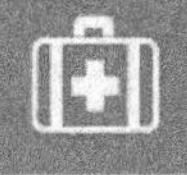

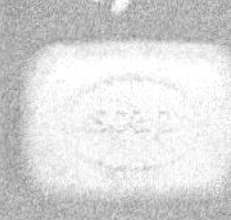

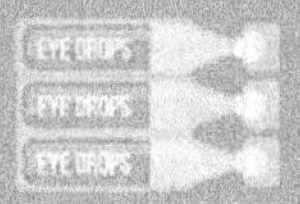

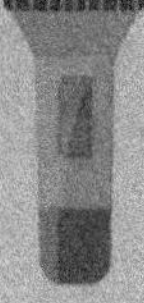

or eyewash solution

Conclusion

Applying basic first aid hacks in various scenarios and situations is a valuable skill that can make a difference in times of need.

In our dynamic world, where accidents and unforeseen emergencies can happen at any time, the ability to apply basic first aid hacks is an invaluable skill. These hacks empower individuals to become the first line of defense providing immediate assistance and potentially saving lives.

In scenarios involving minor injuries, knowing how to stop bleeding, treat burns, or alleviate insect stings can provide immediate relief. When faced with more severe situations, such as cardiac arrest, choking, or allergic reactions, applying CPR, the Heimlich maneuver, or using an epinephrine auto-injector can be life-saving acts.

NB: This book focuses more on the basic home first aid guide everyone needs to have. If you wish to learn more about basic first aid, make sure to check out my book " Basic first aid guide" on Amazon.

But remember, first aid hacks are not a substitute for professional medical care, and knowing when to seek professional help is just as important as knowing how to apply first aid. Always prioritize safety, and in serious or uncertain situations, don't hesitate to call 911 or your local emergency number.

As you continue to explore the world of first aid hacks, make it a point to stay updated on the latest techniques and guidelines through first aid training and certifications. Your commitment to preparedness and the application of these skills not only benefits you but also those around you, contributing to a safer and more resilient community. Embrace the power of first aid hacks and be ready to face life's unexpected challenges with confidence and resourcefulness. Your knowledge can make all the difference in someone's time of need.

Enjoyed Our Book? Share Your Thoughts with the World!

Dear Unique Responder

I hope this message finds you well, and I want to express my sincere gratitude for choosing to read and learn from my book, **"Basic First Aid Hacks"**. Your support means the world to me, and I'm thrilled that you've taken this journey with me through the pages of my work.

If you enjoyed reading, gained additional knowledge from **"Basic First Aid Hacks"** and found it valuable, I kindly request you to consider leaving a review on Amazon. Your review will not only be a great source of encouragement for me but will also help other potential readers discover the book.

Sharing your thoughts about the book, whether it's your favorite parts, what home remedies you never knew were at your reach, or how it may have positively impacted your life, can make a significant difference. Honest reviews from readers like you play a crucial role in the success of a book, and they serve as a guide for others seeking their next educational read.

Here's how to leave a review on Amazon:

- [ ] Visit the Amazon website and log in to your Amazon account.
- [ ] Search for **"Basic First Aid Hacks"** in the Amazon search bar.
- [ ] Click on the book's title to go to the book's page.
- [ ] Scroll down to the "Customer Reviews" section.
- [ ] Click the "Write a customer review" button.
- [ ] Share your thoughts, rating, and any insights you have about the book.
- [ ] Click "Submit" to post your review.

Your feedback is incredibly valuable to me, and it helps me improve. Plus, it lets other readers know what they can expect from **"Basic First Aid Hacks."**

Once again, thank you for choosing to read my book, and I appreciate your support.

Wishing you many more wonderful growth as you forge ahead with **Basic First Aid Hacks!**

Thank you!

First Aid for Cardiac Arrest
Emergency Treatment

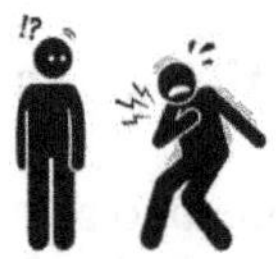

Cardiac Arrest

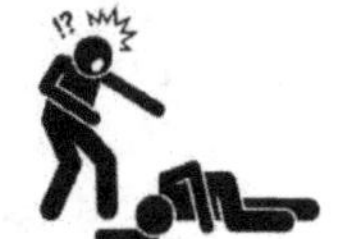

Victim Collapses

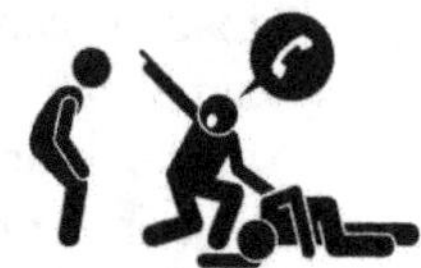

Ask for Help

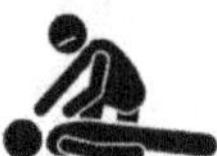

Check Vital Signs

Check Breathing

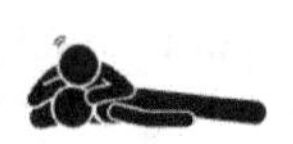

Rescue Breath

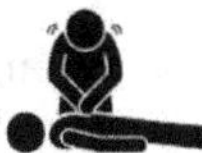

Perform CPR

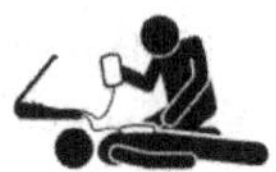

Use AED

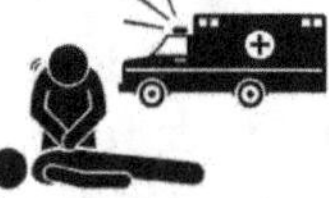

Wait for Ambulance

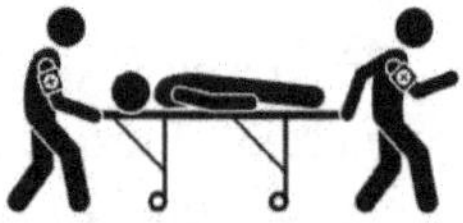

Send Victim to Hospital

First Aid for Choking

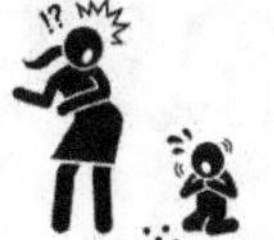

Choking

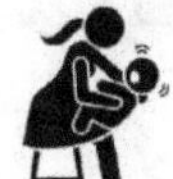

Check Mouth

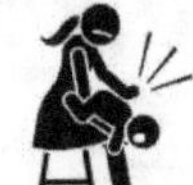

Back Blows

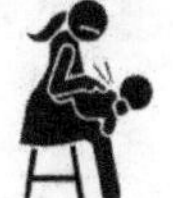

Chest Thrust

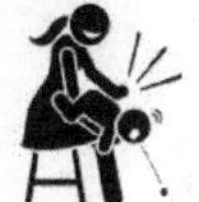

Cough up Object

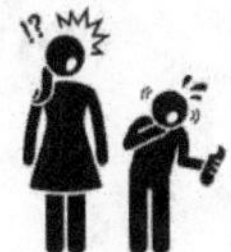

Choking

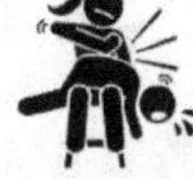

Back Blows

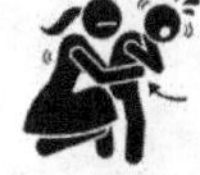

Abdominal Thrust

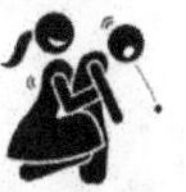

Cough up Object

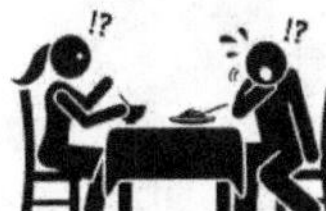

Choking

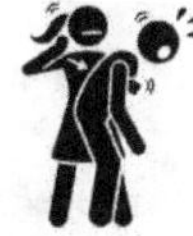

Back Blows

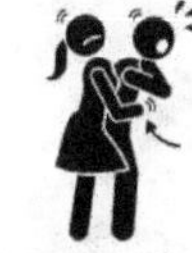

Abdominal Thrust

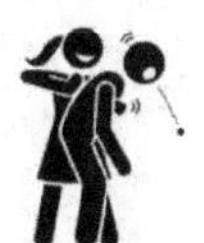

Cough Up Object

ABCs of First Aid

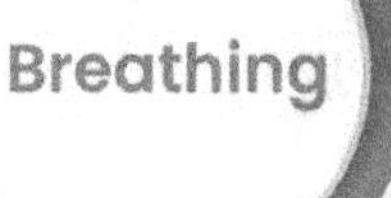

If someone's not breathing, clear their airway

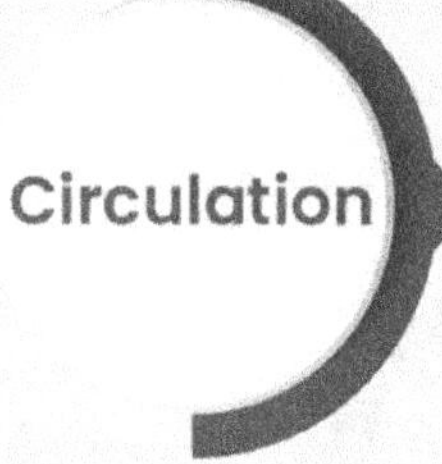

If the airway is clear and they're still not breathing, provide rescue breathing

Perform chest compressions to keep blood circulating, as well as rescue breathing. If the person is breathing but unresponsive, check their pulse. If their heart has stopped, provide chest compressions